Whole Food and Plant Based Diet a 28 day plan

Table of Contents

Introduction

Whole foods plant based diets means not only taking fruit and vegetables. This Diet is Good for your Body and have some different from vegetarian diet. Also good for your skin and environment and majority of this food you eat comes from whole which is unprocessed food. Although, some little amount of lean meat and fish is allow in this diet. But eating plant based foods is the main target. Whole foods should be close to the original basis as much as possible.

A whole foods diet can prevent the risk of diabetes, hypertension and heart disease not only that it can help you lose weight. It can give you attractive skin and can keep your your digestive system normal. When you will follow the right diet you will get all of such amazing benefits.

Not only for these type of disease can you consider whole foods to lose weight and beautiful skin. There are no committed rules that you must follow and no risk of failing the diet. When you put your best foot forward and choose the right foods to eat on a regular basis, your health will benefit

I hope, this book will help you to accustom with new diet plans. I hope, you will love this Book recipe and you will follow this diet.

Chapter 1: What is the Whole Food and Plant Based Diet?

To follow this whole food diet at first you have to understand what whole foods is plant based diet means. Simply, whole food plant based diet is a foods that are filled a majority of foods that are not processed or refined and come from plats directly. This foods are completely unmodified and close to their original source. It is not a diet limited only to fruits and vegetables; there are many delightful options to aid you have a satisfying choice of foods to eat.

They are not processed and have little to no extracts including sugar, salt and artificial elements. These foods are raw and can be eaten in their natural condition. They need little to no changes, which is why you are able to increase the advantage of close to 100 percent of the vital nutrients that the food has to offer. Whole foods decrease the likelihood of losing the vital nutrients in each type of food that happens when they are processed or even in some ways of cooking.

Chapter 2: Breakfast Recipes

MORNING POWER GREEN SMOOTHIE

Ingredients:

- 2 Bananas, peeled and frozen
- 1 Apple, minced
- 1 cup Kale, minced
- 2 cups Almond milk, unsweetened
- 2 tablespoons Nut butter (whichever you like)
- 1 teaspoon Vanilla bean powder (optional)
- 1 teaspoon Cinnamon
- 1 tablespoon Chia seeds
- A few ice cubes (not necessary)

Instructions:

1. Mix together in a blender: almond milk, oats, kale and frozen bananas. Puree.

2. As soon as they are pureed add in apple slices and continue blending till smooth again.

3. Add in nut butter, vanilla bean powder, cinnamon, and chia seeds. Run blender until you make a perfect smoothie and enjoy its great taste!

GRATED BANANA COCONUT PANCAKES

Ingredients:

- 4 Eggs
- ½ cup Coconut flour
- 2 Bananas, grated
- 1 teaspoon Baking Soda
- ½ teaspoon Cinnamon, ground
- 1½ tablespoon Coconut oil
- 1 tablespoon Coconut flakes
- ½ cup Bilberries or your favorite berries
- 3 tablespoon Coconut sugar (exclude for Paleo)

Instructions:

1. Beat up the eggs in the bowl and add coconut flour, grated bananas, soda, and cinnamon and coconut sugar (exclude sugar if you are doing paleo). Continue whisking until smooth.

2. Heat up the frying pan with ½ tablespoon coconut oil.

3. Ladle the batter to the pan, so that you make 4 or 5 small pancakes.

4. Cook and flip the pancakes as soon as you see bubbles on its upper surface.

5. When the pancakes are ready, take them off the pan into the large plate. Put ½ tablespoon more coconut oil to the pan and repeat steps 3-5.

6. Cover pancakes, making sure they stay hot until you are done with the others.

7. Sprinkle the pancakes with the coconut flakes and garnish with your favorite berries, such as .bilberries, raspberries, etc., or their mix.

8. Serve hot banana coconut pancakes immediately.

SPROUTED BUCKWHEAT, FRESH BERRIES, AND COCONUT YOGURT

Ingredients:

- ½ cup sprouted and dehydrated Buckwheat, organic
- ½ cup organic Coconut yogurt
- 2 tablespoons Goji berries
- 1 cup fresh Blueberries/Blackberries/Raspberries/Cherries or their mix
- 1 ½ tablespoons Hemp seeds
- 1 ½ tablespoons Pumpkin seeds, sprouted
- 1 teaspoon Cinnamon
- 1 teaspoon Turmeric
- 1 teaspoon Vanilla extract
- 1 pinch of Sea salt

Instructions:

1. Soak goji berries in warm water for about 10 minutes before you start.

2. Place dehydrated sprouted buckwheat to the serving bowl. Cover it with coconut yogurt.

3. Add your favorite berries, hemp seeds, pumpkin seeds and goji berries. Sprinkle your salad with salt, cinnamon, turmeric and vanilla. Enjoy!

SWEET POTATO & BROCCOLI VEGETARIAN PATTIES

Ingredients:

- 1 Sweet potato (yam), medium-sized
- 1 cup Broccoli heads
- 1 Egg
- 1 cup Breadcrumbs
- ½ cup White cheddar cheese, grated
- 1 Green onion, minced
- 1 tablespoon Extra virgin olive oil
- Smoked paprika, ground pepper, sea salt and garlic powder to taste

Instructions:

1. Steam potato until fork tender.

2. Steam broccoli. It's the most convenient to use the pot with steamer.

3. Use potato masher or fork to make sweet potato puree and add shredded steamed broccoli, 3 tablespoons bread crumbs, egg, white cheddar, green onion and all spices to taste. Mix very well.

4. Scoop 2 tablespoons of this "dough" and roll a veggie ball in your palm. Do the same with all of the mixture. You should be able to make 10-12 patties with this amount of ingredients.

5. Dip the balls in the rest of breadcrumbs and squeeze between your palms to make patties.

6. Heat the olive oil in the skillet and put the patties to cook for 3-4 minutes each side.

FRUITY CREAMY ANTI-PIZZA

Ingredients:

- 1 fresh-cut slice Watermelon, diameter 10-inches or so
- 2 Apricots, seeded and sliced
- 1 Nectarine, sliced
- 5-7 large Strawberries, halved
- 5-7 large Raspberries
- ½ cup Blueberries
- 2 tablespoons + 2 tablespoons (separately) Honey
- ½ cup Heavy cream
- A few leaves of Mint

Instructions:

1. Whip refrigerated heavy cream on medium-high speed with the help of a mixer. It may take 2-3 minutes to make it thick.

2. Switch mixer's speed to the lowest and whisk in 2 tablespoons of honey. Continue whisking for 2 more minutes.

3. Evenly cover large watermelon slice with prepared cream. Place apricots, nectarine, strawberries, raspberries and blueberries on top of it. Drizzle berries and fruits with remaining 2 honey tablespoons.

4. Sprinkle pizza with mint leaves and divide into slices. Enjoy this piece of culinary art!

HALF-HOUR MUFFIN FRITTATAS

Ingredients:

- 1 large Red bell pepper, minced
- ¾ cup Zucchini, minced

- 2 tablespoons Red onion, minced
- 6 Eggs
- 1 cup Cheddar cheese, shredded
- ½ cup organic Milk
- ¼ tablespoon Sea salt
- Chile pepper to taste
- Ground Black pepper to taste

Instructions:

1. Preheat oven to 350 F.

2. Break eggs in the bowl. Add milk, black pepper, chile pepper and salt. Mix well until you make the mixture perfectly smooth.

3. Add minced zucchini, onion, and red bell pepper. Stir thoroughly.

4. You will now need to use muffin cups or nonstick muffin pan. Add the mixture into muffin cups or nonstick muffin pan with the help of a spoon. 4-5 spoons of the mixture should be enough to cover it completely.

5. Bake for about 20 minutes and transfer muffin frittatas to a wire rack to chill for 5 minutes. Remove muffin frittatas from cups or muffin pan. Serve.

SPINACH TOMATO-FETA WHITE OMELETTE

Ingredients:

- 3 Egg whites
- 5 tablespoons Spinach, freshly chopped
- 6 Cherry tomatoes, sliced
- 2 tablespoons Feta cheese

- 1 teaspoon Extra virgin olive oil
- Sea salt and ground pepper to taste

Instructions:

1. Oil the frying pan and put it on the medium heat.

2. Separate egg whites and whisk them with the sea salt and black pepper.

3. Pour the mixture into the heated pan and cook for 2 minutes.

4. Add feta, spinach and cherry tomatoes in the middle and cook for 2 more minutes.

5. Fold omelet in half with the help of a turner. Cook until feta cheese is molten for about 2 more minutes. Serve immediately.

SUPER FRUIT & NUT SALAD ON TOP OF BROWN RICE WITH CACAO PUREE

Ingredients:

- 1 ½ cups Brown rice, pre-cooked
- 1 tablespoon Coconut sugar, melted
- 1 Banana, peeled and minced
- 2 Kiwis, peeled and minced
- 2 Tangerines, peeled and minced
- 1 tablespoon Goji berries
- 2 tablespoons Lemon juice
- ½ teaspoon Tangerine or Lemon zest
- 1 tablespoon + 3 tablespoons (separately) Walnuts, raw
- 5 tablespoons Cashew nuts, raw
- 1 tablespoon Agave syrup

- 2 tablespoons Cacao powder
- 1 cup Water

Instructions:

1. Soak cashew nuts and walnuts for at least 1 hour in hot water. Drain. This will help you to blend the nuts later. It's especially important to do if you do not have a food processor or high-speed blender. If you do have any of those, you may skip this step.

2. Pre-cook brown rice and stir in melted coconut sugar. Cover it and let it stay warm.

3. In a large bowl combine banana, kiwis, tangerines, goji berries, 1 tablespoon walnuts, zest and sprinkle with lemon juice. Toss fruit salad thoroughly. Put it into the refrigerator to chill.

4. Put into the food processor or high-speed blender the ingredients for cacao cream including water, cacao powder, soaked cashew nuts and 3 tablespoons walnuts and agave syrup. Blend until you get ideal cacao-nut puree.

5. Transfer some brown rice into the bottom of the serving bowl. Cover the rice with some cocoa puree. Put on top of it chilled super fruit salad. Serve.

MANGO MELON FRESH SALAD

Ingredients:

- 1 cup Blueberry, halved
- 3 cups Casaba (honeydew) melon, peeled, bite-size minced
- 1 cup Yellow mango, ripe, peeled and minced
- 2 Limes, freshly squeezed

- 1 tablespoon Coconut sugar
- ½ cup Mint leaves, fresh
- ½ teaspoon Cinnamon, ground

Instructions:

1. In a small pan melt quickly 1 tablespoon of Coconut sugar.

2. Mix up in the large bowl fresh mint leaves, halved blueberries, minced casaba melon, and ripe yellow mango. Pour freshly squeezed juice of limes and melted coconut sugar. Stir thoroughly.

3. Sprinkle with cinnamon and serve.

CLASSIC GRANOLA WITH FRESH FRUITS AND BERRIES

Ingredients:

- 1 ½ cups Granola
- 1 Banana, chopped
- ½ cup Blueberries, fresh
- ½ cup Raspberries, fresh
- 1 tablespoon Coconut flakes
- Handful of Cashews roasted without salt
- 1 teaspoon Almonds, chopped
- 1 cup Milk, whole

Instructions:

1. Split granola within 2 bowls.

2. Add fresh banana, blueberries, raspberries, almonds, cashews, coconut flakes, and pour milk.

3. Fresh blueberries and raspberries may be replaced with fresh blackberries and strawberries. You may experiment with your favorite berries. Ripe yellow mango also tastes great with this classic granola.

ALMOND BANANA CREAMY PUDDING

Ingredients:

- 4 tablespoons Almond butter
- 4 tablespoons Almonds, crushed
- 1 can Coconut milk (13.5 oz.)
- 1 tablespoon Coconut sugar
- 1 Banana, overripe

Instructions:

1. Open coconut milk can without prior shaking. Separate the coconut water from the cream. You won't need the water for this recipe, but most likely you would like to keep it and to use it for something else, e.g. cocktails, smoothies, bakery, etc.

2. Combine coconut cream with melted coconut sugar and whisk with a mixer until you get a coconut milk whipped cream.

3. Remove 1 tablespoon of whipped cream and put aside in a small saucer.

4. Take the bowl with the most part of whipped cream and add almond butter and banana. Continue whisking until the mixture is perfectly smooth.

5. The creamy pudding is ready, so transfer it to the serving dish. Add on top 1 tablespoon of whipped cream that you have put aside in step 3. Sprinkle the pudding with crushed almonds.

AVOCADO OMELET WITH CHEDDAR AND RED BELL PEPPER

Ingredients:

- 3 Eggs
- 3 tablespoons whole Milk
- 6 tablespoons Cheddar cheese, grated
- 1 Avocado, peeled, deseeded and diced
- ¼ cup Red bell pepper, diced
- 1 tablespoon Green onion, chopped
- 1 teaspoon Olive oil

Instructions:

1. Break the eggs, pour in milk and whisk.

2. Heat the olive oil in a large nonstick frying pan.

3. Set medium-low heat. Pour in milk-egg mixture and cook it until omelet top is nearly set.

4. Continue cooking as you sprinkle omelet with green onion and grated cheddar. In 2 more minutes, the cheese should melt. Turn off the heat.

5. Now sprinkle omelet with the cubes of avocado and bell pepper. Fold in half and serve.

GRANOLA CRUST FRUIT-N-BERRY PIZZA

Ingredients:

- 1 cup + 1 ½ tablespoons (separately) Granola
- ½ cup Coconut yogurt
- ½ cup Coconut, shredded
- ½ cup dried Raisins
- ½ cup dried Cherries
- ½ cup Purple grapes, halved
- ½ cup Pichuberries, halved
- 2 tablespoons Pomegranate seeds
- 2 tablespoons Coconut oil

Instructions:

1. Mix up coconut yogurt and shredded coconut and let it stand aside and soften.

2. Mix 1 cup granola, raisins, and dried cherries. Add in coconut oil. Pulse in a food processor until you get a rough dough. Shape "pizza template" on a serving plate and put it into the fridge to chill for at least 15 minutes.

3. Drizzle pizza template with coconut mixture and cover it with halved grapes, pichuberries and pomegranate seeds. Sprinkle fruit and berry pizza with remaining 1 ½ tablespoons of granola. Refrigerate and serve.

CINNAMON APPLE SLICES

Ingredients:

- 2 lb. Apples, peeled and sliced

- 6 tablespoons Brown sugar
- 1 tablespoon Coconut oil
- 1 pinch Nutmeg
- 1 teaspoon Cinnamon, powdered
- 2 tablespoons Water

Instructions:

1. Mix up together sliced apples, cinnamon, nutmeg and brown sugar.

2. Take a medium saucepan and combine coconut oil, water, and the mixture from the step 1.

3. Cook at medium heat stirring from time to time for 9-10 minute until apples become fork tender.

PUREED BERRY OAT BOWL

Ingredients:

- ⅓ cup gluten-free Oats
- 1 Banana, ripe
- ½ cup + 1 tablespoon (separately) Raspberry
- ½ cup Blueberry
- 2 tablespoons Goji berries
- 1 tablespoon Blackberry
- 3 tablespoons Chia seeds
- 1 tablespoon Pumpkin seeds
- 4 tablespoons + ½ cup (separately) Coconut milk

Instructions:

1. In a mason jar combine 4 tablespoons of coconut milk with chia seeds and oats. Shake and leave in the fridge overnight.

2. Just before breakfast combine ½ cup of blueberries, ½ cup of raspberries, ½ cup of coconut milk, ripe banana and chilled oat mixture. Blend to make a smooth oat berry puree.

3. Transfer pureed berry oat mix to the serving bowl and sprinkle it with goji berries, pumpkin seeds, blackberries and remaining 1 tablespoon of raspberries. Ready to eat!

BROWN RICE BLUEBERRY HOT CEREAL

Ingredients:

- 1 cup Brown rice, cooked
- 1 cup whole Milk
- 1 Egg
- 1 tablespoon Natural honey
- ½ cup dried Blueberries
- 2-3 walnuts, shredded
- 1 dash Cinnamon
- 1 pinch Vanilla extract

Instructions:

1. Put the cooked brown rice into a medium-sized saucepan and add whole milk, dried blueberries, honey, and cinnamon. Bring to the boil and simmer for 20 minutes at the slow heat.

2. Stir the broken egg in the cup and slowly stir in about 5 teaspoons of hot cereal from the saucepan.

3. Add the mixture of egg and cereal from the cup to the saucepan.

4. Add vanilla extract, stir thoroughly and cook for 2-3 more minutes.

5. Add walnuts and serve warm.

CHEESY POTATO CHICKEN SPINACH BREAKFAST HASH

Ingredients:

- 1 Potato, peeled and minced
- ½ lb. Chicken breast, pre-cooked and finely minced
- 2 Eggs
- 1 cup + ½ cup (separately) Cheddar, shredded
- 4 tablespoons Milk, organic
- 2 tablespoons Butter, melted
- 3 tablespoons + 1 tablespoon (separately) Olive oil
- 1 Onion, small and finely minced
- 1 cup Baby spinach, minced roughly
- 2 tablespoons + 1 tablespoon (separately) Green onion, finely minced
- 1 tablespoon Cilantro leaves, minced
- Sea salt, paprika and ground black pepper to taste

Instructions:

1. Heat 3 tablespoons olive oil in a large skillet over medium-low heat. Add in onion and potato. Sprinkle it with sea salt, paprika, and ground black pepper. Cook it for 10 minutes stirring often. Remove it to a plate to stop the cooking process.

2. Take a large bowl and mix up minced chicken, cilantro, 2 tablespoons green onion, spinach and melted butter. Stir in potato-onion mix.

3. Whisk the eggs and milk. Pour the mixture into the bowl with potato-chicken, add in shredded cheese and toss very well.

4. Grease baking dish with 1 tablespoon olive oil. Transfer the "dough" to the baking dish and press softly. Sprinkle it with another ½ cup shredded cheddar. Cover the baking dish with tinfoil.

5. Let the baking dish with all prepared ingredients sit for 20-30 minutes. In the meanwhile preheat oven to 375 F.

6. Bake this breakfast hash for 20 minutes covered with tinfoil, and then 20 minutes uncovered. As soon as it is ready and removed from the oven, sprinkle it with remaining 1 tablespoon green onion and let it sit for 10 minutes. Serve the breakfast hash hot or chilled.

TOMATO AVOCADO TOAST

Ingredients:

- 2 slices Whole meal bread, toasted
- 2 ½ tablespoons Cilantro, minced
- 5 Cherry tomatoes, minced
- 1 Avocado, peeled, seeded, pureed
- 1 tablespoon Olive oil
- Pinch of Oregano
- Ground Pepper and Salt to taste

Instructions:

1. Combine pureed avocado with olive oil and cilantro. Mix thoroughly and spread toasted whole meal bread with this avocado mix.

2. Top the toast with cherry tomatoes and sprinkle with ground pepper, oregano, and salt.

STRAWBERRY-MILLET BOWL

Ingredients:

- 1 lb. Strawberries
- 1 cup Millet
- 1 cup Milk + 1 cup fresh Water (mixed)
- 3 tablespoons Milk (separately)
- 1 tablespoon Honey
- 1 tablespoon extra-virgin olive oil
- 2 tablespoons Pistachios, finely chopped
- 4 sticks Thyme
- 1 ½ teaspoon Vanilla
- Handful Hemp seeds

Instructions:

1. Preheat oven to 450 F.

2. Halve strawberries and mix them up with honey, thyme, and olive oil. Transfer them to a baking sheet and bake until strawberries start releasing its juice. It may take 8-12 minutes. Remove the sheet from the oven and discard thyme sticks. Set the sheet aside.

3. Meanwhile, bring to a boil milk-water mixture and stir in millet with vanilla extract. Make heat low and cover the saucepan. Simmer for 20-30 minutes, until the liquid absorbs and millet is cooked.

4. Transfer millet to a serving bowl; add remaining 3 tablespoons of milk, berries, and juices from the baking sheet. Sprinkle your breakfast bowl with hemp seeds and chopped pistachios.

PEAR ICEBERG FETA SALAD

Ingredients:

- ½ head Iceberg lettuce
- 2 Pears, ripe, sweet and large
- 8 tablespoons Feta cheese
- Handful of Pinenuts
- Handful of Walnuts
- Handful of Raisins
- 8 tablespoons Balsamic vinegar salad dressing

Instructions:

1. Chop iceberg lettuce and pears casually and mix in the salad bowl.

2. Add crumbled feta cheese.

3. Add raisins, walnuts and peanuts, pour vinegar and mix.

4. You may serve the salad immediately or keep covered in the refrigerator for up to 60 minutes before serving.

5. You may try mixing 2 different sorts of pears, e.g. Asian pear and bosc pear are a good combination.

6. You may replace peanuts and raisins with chopped almonds and dried cranberries - it also tastes great!

PUMPKIN PANCAKES

Ingredients:

- 5 Egg whites
- 5 tablespoons Canned pumpkin puree, organic

- 4 tablespoons Whole oats
- 3 tablespoons Cottage cheese
- 1 serving Vanilla whey powder
- ¼ teaspoon Pumpkin pie spice
- ½ teaspoon Vanilla extract
- ½ teaspoon Cinnamon, ground
- 2 tablespoons of Sour cream
- Handful of Bilberries per person
- Pinch of Sea salt

Instructions:

1. Combine all ingredients except plain yogurt and whisk in the large bowl to make the batter.

2. Heat up a nonstick frying pan at medium heat level.

3. Pour the batter in small portions and get the shape of pancakes that you prefer.

4. Flip pancakes when they get light brown and cook for 1-2 more minutes at the other side. Make sure they are finely cooked but not burnt.

5. Transfer pancakes to a large serving bowl and repeat the steps 3 and 4 until you run out of the batter.

6. Serve with sour cream and bilberries.

Chapter 3: Lunch Recipes

AVOCADO-SHRIMP SALAD

Ingredients:

- 2 Avocados, cut into large cubes
- 1 lb. Shrimp, cooked
- 2 Tomatoes, chopped
- 1 small Onion, shredded
- 2 tablespoons Lime juice, fresh
- ½ teaspoon Garlic powder
- ½ small batch of Parsley, chopped
- 1 pinch of Salt
- 1 pinch of Black pepper

Instructions:

1. Mix avocados, shrimp, tomatoes, and onion in a salad bowl.
2. Add salt, pepper, garlic powder, parsley and stir.
3. Season with fresh lime juice.
4. Serve this refreshing salad immediately.

CALAMARI WITH PARSLEY AND GARLIC

Ingredients:

- 1 lb. Squid

- 2.5 tablespoons Extra virgin olive oil
- 1 tablespoon Garlic, chopped
- 1 tablespoon Italian parsley, chopped
- 1 Lemon
- Sea salt and ground pepper to taste

Instructions:

1. Clean and dry the squid with a paper towel. Chop the squid body into ¾ inch-thick rings. Leave tentacles whole.

2. Heat the olive oil in a large pan or wok on the high heat. Add the squid in a single layer and sprinkle with finely chopped garlic, pepper, salt and Italian parsley.

3. Cook constantly mixing for 1 or 2 minutes.

4. Cut lemon wedges to garnish and serve immediately.

EGGPLANT BOATS STUFFED WITH GROUND BEEF

Ingredients:

- 3 lbs. Italian eggplants
- 1½ lbs. Beef, ground
- 1 ½ cups Tomato sauce, organic or homemade
- 1 Onion, large and minced
- 6 cloves Garlic, minced
- 2 ½ tablespoons Extra virgin olive oil
- Handful of Parsley, chopped
- Salt and ground pepper to taste
- ⅓ cup Breadcrumbs (exclude for the Whole30 and Paleo compatibility)

Instructions:

1. Cut eggplants into two parts each and scoop them out. Do not discard eggplant's natural stuffing - put it aside. Grease cleaned out eggplant halves with a bit of olive oil, salt, and pepper.

2. Cover the baking dish with the tin-foil. Put the eggplant "boats" violet color down, white-green color up, so that you will be able to put stuffing inside the "boats" later.

3. Mince eggplant's natural stuffing in the food processor or chop finely. We will need only 2 cups of this mincemeat. You can get rid of the rest.

4. Heat up the frying pan with 1 tablespoon of olive oil. Add 2 cups of eggplant's natural stuffing, minced onion, black pepper and salt. Cook for 7 minutes at medium-high heat and stir from time to time. Add garlic, stir and cook for 1 more minute.

5. Add ground beef to the onion-eggplant mixture and stir thoroughly. Cook for 7 minutes till most of the pink color is gone.

6. Put the frying pan contents to the colander and press out excess fat and liquid.

7. Put the beef-onion-eggplant mixture back to the frying pan and add homemade pasta sauce. Stir and cook for 2 minutes.

8. Remove the mixture from the pan and stuff the eggplant-"boats" with it tightly. Make sure not to overfill the "boats".

9. Preheat oven to 350 F

10. Sprinkle the "boats" with bread crumbs, if you are not following whole30 or paleo program. Add salt, and pepper. Pour a bit of olive oil on top.

11. Bake for 50-60 minutes till eggplant is tender. Remove from oven and let it cool for 10 minutes before consuming.

SIMPLE CHICKEN AND BROCCOLI

Ingredients:

- 7 cups Broccoli flower clusters
- 2 lbs. Chicken, finely minced
- 3 tablespoons Sesame oil, toasted
- ⅔ cup Coconut aminos
- 2 tablespoons Ginger, finely grated
- 1 teaspoon Red pepper flakes
- 1 teaspoon Garlic powder
- 1 teaspoon Sea salt

Instructions:

1. Heat up sesame oil in a large skillet and add broccoli. Sprinkle with garlic powder, grated ginger, red pepper flakes, salt and add coconut aminos. Cook for 5 minutes at medium heat till broccoli is dark green and moderately soft.

2. Switch heat to high. Add chicken and continue cooking constantly stirring for 5 minutes.

3. Serve hot.

4. This chicken and broccoli comply with whole and whole30 diets. It is good to serve it separately or with cauliflower rice and spiralized zucchini noodles.

TWENTY-MINUTE HALIBUT SALAD

Ingredients:

- 5 oz. Halibut fillets
- ½ lb. Salad greens, chopped
- 1 cup Vegetable broth
- 1 Tomato, cubed
- 4 cloves Garlic
- 1 small Onion, chopped
- 1 tablespoon + 4 tablespoons Lemon juice, freshly squeezed
- 3 teaspoons Sage, dried
- 2 tablespoons Extra virgin olive oil
- Salt and ground pepper to taste

Instructions:

1. Take 4 cloves of garlic and crush with a garlic press or mince with the knife. Let it sit and oxidize for 5 minutes as it will get more healthy properties.

2. Rub the fish with 1 tablespoon of freshly squeezed lemon juice and sprinkle with some salt and ground pepper to taste.

3. Bring to boil vegetable broth in a medium bowl and add the fish. Simmer for 10 minutes.

4. In the meanwhile take a salad spinner to wash and dry salad greens. Chop it a little bit and let it sit in four serving plates. Add chopped onion, tomato and stir. As soon as halibut fillets are cooked, simply transfer them from the bowl on top of greens and veggies.

5. We won't need vegetable broth anymore in this recipe. But you may want to keep it if you plan to cook the soup as well. Anyway, remove broth from the bowl, and use the same bowl again to combine pressed or minced garlic, 4 tablespoons of fresh lemon

juice and sage. Heat stirring for half-minute. Turn off the heat and stir in olive oil. Mist it over the salad and halibut.

6. Add more salt and ground pepper if desired.

CURRIED APPLE TUNA WRAPS

Ingredients:

- 3 ½ tablespoons Mayonnaise, organic or homemade
- 6 oz. can Tuna
- 1 large Carrot, grated
- 1 medium Green apple, cubed
- ¼ Red onion, finely chopped
- 1 tablespoon fresh Lemon juice
- 1 teaspoon Curry powder
- 1 tablespoon fresh Parsley, minced
- ½ teaspoon Turmeric
- 1 Collard green leaf, large
- Pinch of salt and ground pepper

Instructions:

1. Combine all ingredients except collard green leaf in a medium bowl and toss very well.

2. Take the collard green leaf and horizontally trim the thick part of its stem. Therefore you will make the stem flat.

3. Transfer tuna apple mixture to the trimmed collard leaf. Fold the leaf sides in and wrap it over itself.

4. Halve the leaf stuffed with apple tuna mixture and put into the serving bowl.

ASIAN SHRIMP AND CAULIFLOWER RICE

Ingredients:

- 8 oz. Shrimp, deveined and peeled
- 1 small head Cauliflower
- 1 Carrot, medium-sized, minced
- 1 Red bell pepper, small, hashed
- 1 cup Onion, hashed
- 2 cloves Garlic, chopped
- 2 Eggs, beaten and mixed
- 1 tablespoon Coconut oil
- Sea salt and ground pepper to taste
- ½ cup Peas (exclude for the Whole30 and Paleo compatibility)

Instructions:

1. Very finely chop cauliflower into so-called "cauliflower rice". It means cauliflower should actually look very close to rice.

2. Heat up large frying pan (ideally wok); add coconut oil, finely chopped onion and garlic. Cook for 3 minutes to make onion soft.

3. Add shrimp to the wok and cook stirring for the other 60 seconds.

4. Add sweet pepper, peas, and carrot and cook for 3 more minutes. Please do not add peas if you are doing the whole30 program or paleo.

5. Add cauliflower rice and stir the way that you have an open circle in the center of your pan.

6. Pour the mixed eggs in the cleared center of your pan, scramble, and then mix up eggs with the rest of the dish. Serve hot.

BELL PEPPER TURKEY NACHOS

Ingredients:

- 1 lb. Turkey, ground
- 4 Bell peppers (the best if you have all different colors)
- 1 Tomato, diced
- 1 medium Onion, minced
- 1 Jalapeno pepper, sliced
- Pace Salsa (sauce from organic food market)
- 3 tablespoons Guacamole
- Handful of green onion, minced
- 1 tablespoon Olive oil
- ½ teaspoon Garlic powder
- ½ teaspoon Cumin powder
- ½ teaspoon Chili powder
- ¼ teaspoon Cayenne pepper
- ½ teaspoon Sea salt

Instructions:

1. Combine diced tomatoes, jalapeno pepper, Pace Salsa and green onion in a medium bowl. Stir and set aside.

2. Mix ground turkey and minced onion with garlic powder, cumin, chili pepper, cayenne pepper and sea salt.

3. Pour olive oil into a large skillet and warm up. Cook ground turkey with species stirring frequently for 8-10 minutes over medium-high heat.

4. Cut bell peppers into bell pepper nachos. Set them as the rays of the sun on a serving plate. Add cooked ground turkey mix in the center.

5. Cover the turkey mix with guacamole. Then put Pace Salsa mixture from the step 1 on top.

6. Eat using whole 30 "nachos" – bell pepper slices.

PINEAPPLE SHRIMP CEVICHE

Ingredients:

- 1 cup Pineapple, minced
- 2 cups Shrimp meat, boiled and minced
- 1 Avocado, minced flesh
- 2 Limes, freshly squeezed
- 1 Red onion, thoroughly minced
- 1 cup Red bell pepper, minced
- ½ batch Cilantro, minced
- 1 clove Garlic, pressed or finely minced
- 1 Chili pepper, small, chopped
- Sea salt and ground pepper to taste

Instructions:

1. Stir thoroughly all ingredients in a ceramic or glass salad bowl. Cover the bowl and chill in the refrigerator.

2. In 1 hour Pineapple Shrimp Ceviche is ready to serve.

CREAMY RED CURRY SLAW

We need to make homemade mayonnaise and cool it down in advance before we can start cooking this meal.

Ingredients:

For Homemade mayonnaise

- 1 Egg, room temperature
- ½ teaspoon Mustard, milled
- 2 tablespoons Apple cider vinegar
- 1 cup and 1 tablespoon Olive oil, light
- ½ teaspoon Sea Salt

For Creamy Red Curry Slaw

- 2 cups Broccoli slaw
- ½ cup Bell pepper, minced
- 1 Avocado, cubed
- 1 tablespoon Thai kitchen red curry
- 4 tablespoons Homemade mayonnaise

Instructions:

1. Add mustard, egg, apple cider vinegar, salt and an egg to the food processor. Whisk for 1 minute. Very slowly add light olive oil. Blend for 1 minute or until the olive oil dissolves completely. Homemade mayonnaise is ready to be put into the refrigerator.

2. Make sure homemade mayonnaise is cooled.

3. Combine cubed avocado, minced bell pepper, broccoli slaw, Thai red curry sauce and homemade mayonnaise. Mix well and enjoy!

SAUTEED SWISS CHARD WITH SLIVERED ALMONDS AND DRIED CHERRIES

Ingredients:

- 1 ¼ lbs. Swiss chard
- 2 Shallots (both green and white parts), chopped thinly

- 5-6 tablespoons Almonds, blanched, split and slivered
- Handful of Dried cherries
- 2 tablespoons + 1 tablespoon (separately) Extra virgin olive oil
- 1 tablespoon Apple cider vinegar
- Sea salt to taste

Instructions:

1. First of all, you need to prepare Swiss chard. Separate stems and leaves with the help of a knife. Chop the stems to ½-inch thick slices. Mince the leaves into large pieces. Set prepared stems and leaves aside separately.

2. Medium-heat the skillet without oil and add almonds. Cook for 3-4 minutes stirring several times. Remove almonds from the pan to stop the cooking process. Let it stand aside.

3. Add 2 tablespoons olive oil to the same skillet and increase heat to medium-high. Add Swiss chard stems and thinly chopped shallots and cook stirring for 5-6 minutes until slightly browned and soft. If it is getting brown too fast, pour in a couple tablespoons water.

4. Continue stirring and add in Swiss chard leaves little by little as they wilt slowly on the pan. Make sure all chard leaves are wilted and remove skillet contents to the large plate.

5. Sprinkle sautéed chard with almonds and dried cherries. Toss and drizzle with 1 tablespoon olive oil and apple cider vinegar.

ARUGULA AND MACKEREL SALAD

Ingredients:

- 1 lb. 5 oz. Mackerel

- Arugula, several leaves
- ½ small batch of Parsley
- 1 Lemon
- 1 Onion, small or medium, sliced
- 1 tcaspoon Capers
- 3 tablespoon Extra virgin olive oil
- Black pepper
- Salt

Instructions:

1. Squeeze ⅔ of the lemon to make a juice.

2. Make seasoning mixing lemon juice and olive oil. Add slices of onion and leave it alone for 15-20 minutes.

3. Wash and clean mackerel and put into boiling salted water for 5 minutes.

4. Separate mackerel meat from all the bones.

5. Put mackerel fillets, arugula, parsley and capers into a deep plate. Season with the mix prepared in step 2 and add black pepper.

6. Serve warm immediately or let it cool in the refrigerator and eat later.

LEMON CHICKEN ZOODLES

Ingredients:

- 4 medium Zucchini, spiralized
- ¼ cup Heavy cream
- 2 Lemons, zest of and juice of
- 1 tablespoon whole Butter

- 2 Chicken breasts, grilled and sliced
- 1 cup + ½ cup (separately) Parmesan, grated
- Sea salt, freshly ground pepper and minced parsley to taste

Instructions:

1. Place spiralized zucchinis into a colander and drain for at least 20 minutes. Cover it with a kitchen towel and squeeze a little bit. This will remove excess water from zucchinis.

2. Prepare lemon sauce by combining heavy cream, lemon juice, 1 cup of parmesan and lemon zest. Sprinkle the mixture with salt and pepper and stir thoroughly. Leave it aside for a while.

3. Heat up butter in a large nonstick skillet and add dried spiralized zucchinis. Cook them stirring frequently for about 3 minutes over medium heat.

4. Switch the heat to low and pour in the lemon sauce. Add the slices of grilled chicken breasts and stir well.

5. Cook for 2 minutes more over medium heat.

6. Turn off the heat and sprinkle with another ½ cup of parmesan cheese and minced parsley.

7. Transfer lemon zoodles to serving plates and serve.

VEGAN RAMEN SOUP WITH ZOODLES

Ingredients:

- 4 cups Vegetable stock
- 1 Zucchini, large, spiralized
- 3.5 oz. Shiitake mushrooms

- 1 medium Yellow onion, slices into four parts
- 1 clove Garlic, minced
- 2 Eschalots, chopped and separated white and green parts
- 7 oz. Baby bok choy, chopped
- Ginger, 1-inch piece, peeled and chopped
- ½ tablespoon Miso paste, yellow or white
- 2 tablespoons Soy sauce, low sodium
- 2 tablespoons Sesame oil
- 1 teaspoon Sesame seeds
- Sea salt and freshly ground pepper to taste

Instructions:

1. Heat up 1 tablespoon of sesame oil in a large skillet. Coat the baby bok choy with miso paste and cook for 3 minutes each side at medium-high heat. Remove from the skillet and place aside.

2. Add 1 more tablespoon of sesame oil to the skillet. Add white eschalots, garlic, onion, ginger, pinch of salt and ground pepper. Cook at the same heat for 5 minutes.

3. Pour in low sodium soy sauce and 4 cups of vegetable stock. Cover the skillet to make the mixture boil fast.

4. Add shiitake mushrooms and switch the heat to low. Simmer for 5 minutes till mushrooms are soft.

5. Add spiralized zucchini noodles and simmer for 3 more minutes.

6. You can use pasta tongs to deliver the noodles from the skillet to the deep plates and ladle for the rest of the soup ingredients.

7. Add baby bok choy cooked in Step 1 directly to the serving plates. Also, garnish with sesame seeds and white eschalots. Add more ground pepper and salt if needed.

FRESH CORN, TOMATO AND MOZZARELLA SALAD

Ingredients:

- 6 ears Corn, fresh
- 8 oz. Mozzarella, cubed
- 2 cups Grape tomatoes, red and/or yellow, halved
- 1 ½ cups Basil, minced
- 1 bunch Eschalot, finely minced both green and white parts
- 3 tablespoons White wine vinegar
- 4 tablespoons Olive oil
- Sea salt and ground pepper to taste

Instructions:

1. Combine and mix up white wine vinegar, a pinch of pepper and 2 teaspoons of sea salt. Whisk in the olive oil little by little in a steady stream. This will help to make a very smooth salad dressing.

2. Take fresh corn ears and a sharp knife. Shear them off over a medium bowl.

3. Add to the same bowl halved tomatoes, eschalot and cubed mozzarella. Stir and pour in the dressing.

4. Cover fresh corn salad and let it stand for 15-120 minutes.

5. Sprinkle the corn salad with minced basil right before serving.

SLOW COOKER CAULIFLOWER SOUP

Ingredients:

- 4 cups Vegetable stock
- 2 lbs. Cauliflower, minced

- 2 cups Milk
- 2 lbs. Sweet potato, peeled and diced
- 6 cloves Garlic, peeled
- 2 medium Onions, cubed
- 1 batch Green onion, minced and split into 2 equal portions
- 1 teaspoon Paprika
- ½ teaspoon Red pepper flakes
- 1 teaspoon Thyme
- 2 oz. Cream cheese
- Sea salt and black pepper to taste

Instructions:

1. You need to have a 5-6 quart slow cooker for this amount of ingredients. Pour in vegetable stock and add potato, cauliflower, garlic, onion, paprika, pepper flakes, thyme, salt and the first portion of green onion. Cover slow cooker and cook at high temperature for 4 hours.

2. Turn off the slow cooker and pour in milk and cream cheese.

3. Blend the soup with the help of immersion blender. You may use the other devices, but this one will be the easiest to use with that amount of soup.

4. Transfer vegetable soup to the serving bowls. You will get about 16 portions. Keep in mind this soup may be stored for 4 days in the refrigerator and for up to 2 months frozen. Please make sure you sprinkle the soup with the last portion of fresh green onions just before consuming it.

PINEAPPLE CARROT RAISIN SALAD

Ingredients:

- 1 lb. Carrots, grated
- ⅓ cup fresh Pineapple, minced
- ½ cup Raisins
- 1 tablespoon Coconut sugar, melted
- ½ cup Mayonnaise, homemade or organic gluten-free

Instructions:

1. Insert raisins to the boiling water and boil them for 5 minutes. This preparation will plump them up. Remove raisins and dry using napkin or paper towel.

2. Combine all 5 ingredients and stir thoroughly. Enjoy your super easy and fast lunch!

ORANGE AND FIG FRISEE SALAD

Ingredients:

- 3 handfuls of Frisée, washed and dried
- 5 Figs, overripe and quartered
- 1 Orange, peeled, deseeded and cut into rounds
- 1 teaspoon Honey/Coconut Sugar
- 1 teaspoon Balsamic vinegar
- Pinch of Sea salt
- Ground Black pepper to taste

Instructions:

1. In a small bowl pour in honey (or melted coconut sugar) and stir in balsamic vinegar. Stir until you get the smooth dressing.

2. Mix up orange rounds, frisée and quartered figs in a medium bowl.

3. Sprinkle orange-fig salad with dressing and season with some pepper and salt. It may be served right away.

MEDITERRANEAN WRAP WITH COUSCOUS

Ingredients:

*   4 Spinach tortillas (homemade or from organic food market)
*   1 lb. Chicken tenders
*   1/3 cup Couscous
*   ½ cup fresh Water
*   2 Cucumbers, minced
*   1 Tomato, minced
*   3 cloves Garlic, crushed
*   ½ cup Mint, very finely minced
*   1 cup Parsley, very finely minced
*   4 tablespoons fresh Lemon juice
*   2 tablespoons + 1 tablespoon (separately) Olive oil
*   Sea salt and ground pepper to taste

Instructions:

1. Stir in couscous into a saucepan with boiling water, cover and take off the heat. Let it saturate with water for 5 minutes and fluff couscous using a fork. Leave it aside.

2. Combine garlic, very finely chopped mint and parsley. Pour in fresh lemon juice and 2 tablespoons of olive oil. Add salt, pepper and stir the mint mixture.

3. Add 1 tablespoon of the mint-parsley mixture into a separate medium bowl and combine with the chicken tenders.

4. Heat up a non-stick skillet with 1 tablespoon of olive oil inside. Place tenders into the skillet and cook over medium heat for 3-5 minutes one side, and 2-4 minutes another side, until cooked. Transfer the chicken tenders to a clean plate and let them chill.

5. Transfer remaining mint-parsley mixture into the bowl with prepared couscous. Stir in minced cucumbers and tomato. Add an equal amount of this new mixture onto each spinach tortilla. There will be about ¾ cups for each wrap.

6. Chicken tenders should be chilled enough now. Place them on the cutting board and cut into half-inch size pieces. Add an equal amount of chicken onto each tortilla. Roll the wraps up and halve them. Serve immediately or chilled.

AMAZING TOMATO SOUP

Ingredients:

- 46 oz. Tomato juice (bottle or can)
- 2 cans Diced tomatoes (2 x 14.5 oz.)
- 1 Yellow or white onion, medium-sized, diced
- 2 tablespoons Chicken base
- 6 tablespoons organic Butter
- 1 ½ cups Heavy cream
- 4 tablespoons Parsley, minced
- 4 tablespoons Basil, minced
- 3-5 tablespoons Brown sugar

- ½ teaspoon ground Black pepper

Instructions:

1. Melt butter in a large cooking pot, add onion and cook over medium heat for 3-4 minutes.

2. Stir in diced tomatoes and add tomato juice.

3. Depending on your taste and acidity of tomatoes (which may be different in their nature) add 3-5 tablespoons brown sugar. Start with 3 tablespoons and add more if needed.

4. Continue cooking at medium heat as you add chicken base and black pepper. Stir thoroughly and wait when it almost boils. Then immediately turn off the heat and stir in heavy cream.

5. Sprinkle with parsley and basil leaves and let it sit covered for at least 20 minutes. Serve warm or chilled.

JICAMA-APPLE WHITE BALSAMIC SALAD

Ingredients:

Main Ingredients:

- 1 Napa cabbage, medium-size, sliced
- 2 Apples, peeled and cubed
- 3 Carrots, grated
- 1 Jicama, large, peeled and cubed
- 1 cup Dried cranberries
- 1 bunch Green onions, chopped, only white parts

Balsamic Dressing Ingredients:

- 7 tablespoons White balsamic vinegar
- 3 tablespoons Extra virgin olive oil
- 3 tablespoons Honey, organic
- 3 tablespoons Dijon mustard
- 4 tablespoons Mayonnaise, homemade or organic
- 12 tablespoons Plain Yogurt
- Fresh juice of 1 Lime
- 3 cloves Garlic, minced
- 1 tablespoon Fennel seeds

Instructions:

1. Take a large bowl and mix the napa cabbage, white parts of green onions, jicama, carrots, apples, and cranberries.

2. Take a smaller bowl and add honey, mustard, olive oil, garlic, vinegar, fresh lime juice, mayonnaise and plain yogurt. Strenuously whisk. Add fennel seeds. The dressing is ready.

3. Pour the dressing into the large bowl with the mixed vegetables, berries and fruits described in step 1. Stir thoroughly.

4. Cover the salad and put into the refrigerator for at least 1 hour before serving.

Chapter 4: Dinner Recipes

BRUSSELS SPROUTS WITH LEMON & SUN-DRIED TOMATOES

Ingredients:

- 1 lb. Brussels sprouts
- ¼ cup Sun-dried tomatoes in oil
- ½ cup fresh Water and 4 tablespoons Lemon juice (mixture)
- 1 tablespoon Olive oil
- 1 teaspoon Dijon mustard (alcohol-free)
- ¼ teaspoon Sea salt
- Pinch of ground black pepper
- 1 teaspoon Arrowroot and 1 tablespoon fresh Water (mixture)

Instructions:

1. Preheat oven to 400 F and cover a baking sheet with tinfoil.

2. Remove sun-dried tomatoes from the oil and chop them.

3. Cut off the bottom of each Brussels sprout. Halve them and put onto the baking sheet. Sprinkle them with olive oil, salt, and ground black pepper and toss thoroughly.

4. Make sure Brussels sprouts rest in a single layer and put them into preheated oven for 20 minutes.

5. Meanwhile, heat up a medium skillet. Add in the water-lemon mixture and drained sun-dried tomatoes. Bring to a boil and quickly stir in arrowroot-water mix. Then add mustard and more pepper and salt to taste. Stir again and if the sauce is too thick, you may want to add 2-4 tablespoons of water and toss the sauce one more time. Cook for 1 minute at low heat and remove the sauce from the skillet.

6. Serve cooked Brussels sprouts covered with 4-5 tablespoons of lemon and sun-dried tomato sauce. Note you will have extra sauce left, so chill it and use later.

BAKED TURKEY BELL PEPPER TACOS

Ingredients:

- 4 Bell peppers, large and brighter to have different colors
- 1 lb. Turkey, ground
- ¾ cup Lettuce, minced
- ¾ cup Tomato, minced
- 1 Onion, minced
- 3 cloves, Garlic, minced
- 2 tablespoons Olive oil
- 2 batches Parsley, chopped
- 1 Lime, cut into wedges
- ½ teaspoon Chili powder
- ¼ teaspoon Cumin, ground
- Salt and ground pepper to taste
- ¾ cup Mozzarella and cheddar cheese mix, shredded (please, avoid it if you are following the Whole30 or Paleo programs)

Instructions:

1. Preheat oven to 400 F.

2. Prepare the filling for bell peppers. Heat up olive oil in the large skillet and add in onion, salt and pepper. Cook stirring occasionally for 2 minutes over medium-high heat. Add in ground turkey, garlic, chili powder, cumin. Cook stirring frequently for 5 minutes. Remove filling to the bowl or large plate to stop the cooking process.

3. Halve each bell pepper vertically and remove all seeds, stem, etc.

4. Bake peppers empty side up for 10 minutes.

5. Remove bell peppers from the oven and insert prepared filling into the peppers.

6. Unless you are following the whole30 or paleo programs, top it with mozzarella-cheddar cheese mix.

7. Sprinkle with parsley. Bake for 10 minutes once again and enjoy!

RED-HOT CHILI SNAPPER

Ingredients:

- 1 can of stewed Tomatoes (14.5 oz.)
- 4 fillets Red snapper (about 6 oz.)
- 1 tablespoon Capers, chopped
- 2 cloves Garlic, minced
- 2 small Chili peppers, cut into 4-5 slices each
- 1 Yellow or white onion, minced
- ½ cup White wine vinegar
- ½ tablespoon Pepper flakes
- 2 tablespoons Extra virgin olive oil
- Sea salt and ground black and red pepper to taste

Instructions:

1. Heat a large skillet with oil over medium heat and add chili peppers, garlic, onion, capers and pepper flakes. Cook until onion is soft.

2. Make heat low and add all contents of stewed tomato can, plus wine vinegar. Simmer for 10-15 minutes, in the meanwhile breaking up tomatoes using a spoon. The sauce must thicken a little bit.

3. Add the snapper fillets into the skillet and push them under the sauce to the skillet bottom. Cover the skillet and simmer fish for 15-20 minutes. Make sure the fillets are cooked pinning them with a fork.

4. Add red pepper to taste if you want it really spicy hot. Garnish with your favorite greens and veggies.

PALEO BEEF FAJITAS

Ingredients:

- 1 ½ lbs. Beef, sliced
- 6 oz. Shiitake mushrooms
- 1 cup Vegetable stock
- 2 Bell peppers (ideally 1 red and 1 green), seeded and minced
- 1 Jalapeno pepper, seeded and minced
- 1 Yellow onion, thinly minced
- 1 clove Garlic, crushed
- 2 tablespoons Coconut oil
- 1 Avocado, seeded, peeled, chopped
- Juice of 1 lime
- 4 tablespoons Cilantro, minced
- 2 handfuls Green onion (green parts only), minced
- ½ teaspoon Oregano
- ¼ teaspoon Cayenne pepper, ground

- ½ teaspoon Chili powder
- ½ teaspoon Salt
- Pinch of Cumin, Black pepper, and Paprika

Instructions:

1. In a large bowl combine meat, fresh juice of lime, chili powder, cayenne pepper, paprika, black pepper, cumin, oregano, and salt. Stir thoroughly.

2. Heat up the coconut oil in the large skillet. Add meat and sear over medium-high heat for 7 minutes, stirring frequently. Remove the meat and set aside, but leave its juices in the skillet.

3. Add the bell peppers, mushrooms, onion, and garlic into the skillet. After 5 minutes of cooking add in vegetable stock, jalapeno pepper, green onion, and stir. Add in prepared meat and stir again. Cook for 6-7 minutes more.

4. Serve garnished with avocado and cilantro.

EGGPLANT MEATBALLS AND TOMATO SAUCE

Ingredients:

- 1 Eggplant, medium-sized, peeled and cubed
- 1 Egg
- 1 tablespoon Almond meal
- 15 oz. Tomato sauce, organic (1 can)
- 1 clove + 2 cloves (separately) Garlic, crushed
- 1 Onion, small, finely chopped
- 2 tablespoons Basil leaves, minced
- 1 teaspoon + 1 teaspoon (separately) Extra virgin olive oil
- 1 teaspoon + 1 tablespoon (separately) classic Italian seasoning

- ½ teaspoon Garlic powder
- ½ teaspoon + ½ teaspoon (separately) Red pepper flakes
- Sea salt and ground pepper to taste

Instructions:

1. Steam or boil peeled and cubed eggplant in a medium bowl for 6-8 minutes until soft. Remove eggplant cubes from the bowl and drain.

2. Preheat oven to 350 F.

3. In another bigger bowl combine pre-cooked eggplants with 1 clove crushed garlic, garlic powder, red pepper flakes, 1 teaspoon olive oil, almond meal, cracked egg, 1 teaspoon Italian seasoning, sea salt and ground pepper to taste. Mix up everything thoroughly and roll out eggplant balls.

4. Cover a baking sheet with parchment paper and place eggplant balls over it. Bake for 15-20 minutes to make them tender.

5. In the meanwhile start cooking tomato sauce. Heat up in a frying pan 2 crushed garlic cloves and 1 teaspoon olive oil and cook stirring for 90 seconds. Stir in onion and continue stirring for 2 more minutes. Add organic tomato sauce from the can, Italian seasoning, and red pepper flakes. Bring to boil and decrease heat to minimal. Simmer for 5 minutes, turn off the heat and leave tomato sauce covered.

6. When the eggplant meatballs are cooked, let them cool a little bit on a plate. Then transfer them into a frying pan with tomato sauce. They are ready to serve in 10 minutes or later. Sprinkle with basil leaves on the serving plate.

7. I garnished eggplant meatballs and tomato sauce with spiralized zucchini noodles. It may be also garnished with cauliflower rice or any other whole diet accompaniment at your choice.

SEARED SALMON WITH SOUR CREAM SAUCE

Ingredients:

- 4 Salmon fillets without bones
- 3 tablespoons Extra virgin olive oil
- Salt and black pepper

Sauce Ingredients:

- 2 tablespoons Sour cream
- 2 tablespoons Mayonnaise, homemade or organic
- 1 tablespoon Dill, fresh and chopped
- 1 tablespoon Chrain, grated
- ⅓ teaspoon Garlic powder
- 1 teaspoon Lemon juice, fresh
- Salt and black pepper

Instructions:

1. Preheat oven to 450 F.

2. Take an oven-safe skillet without plastic handles. Add olive oil and make it hot on the cooking stove, while the oven is getting hot.

3. Sprinkle fish fillets with salt and pepper and put into the skillet with hot olive oil. If the fillets have the skin, put them skin side up.

4. Cook them on the hot plate - one side for 3 minutes. Do not flip to the other side.

5. Transfer the oven-safe skillet from the hot plate into the oven without flipping the fish. Cook for 8-9 minutes.

6. In the meanwhile, you can make the sauce. Blend all sauce ingredients well with the spoon or blender.

7. Remove salmon from the oven and pour the sauce on top of it. Use some more dill for decoration.

8. Seared salmon with sour cream sauce is good to be served with fresh vegetables (lettuce, sliced tomatoes, and cucumbers).

ZUCCHINI NOODLES WITH TOMATO MUSHROOMS

Ingredients:

- 3 lbs. Zucchini, spiralized
- 10 oz. Champignons, chopped
- 1 Yellow onion, medium-sized, chopped
- 14.5 oz. can Diced tomatoes, organic, undrained
- 8 oz. Tomato sauce, organic
- ¼ + ¼ teaspoons Garlic powder
- 1 + 1 tablespoons Extra virgin olive oil
- 1 tablespoon Balsamic vinegar
- Freshly ground pepper to taste

Instructions:

1. Heat up 1 tablespoon olive oil in a large saucepan over medium-high heat. Add button mushrooms, yellow onion and cook stirring from time to time for 5 minutes.

2. Add ¼ teaspoon garlic powder, freshly ground pepper, tomato sauce, vinegar, undrained diced tomatoes and bring to boil. Switch the heat to low and simmer. Stir a few times while it is simmering for 9-10 minutes.

3. Take a large skillet with heated up another 1 tablespoon of olive oil. Add zucchini noodles, another ¼ teaspoon Garlic powder, and cook stirring at medium-high heat for 4-5 minutes.

4. Serve zucchini noodles topped with tomato-mushroom sauce.

GRILLED LEMON CHICKEN SKEWERS AND CHERRY TOMATOES

Ingredients:

- 4 Chicken breasts, 1-inch size pieces cubed
- 20-25 Cherry tomatoes
- 7 cloves + 2 cloves (separately) Garlic, crushed
- Juice and zest of 2 Lemons (each lemon separately)
- 1 Lemon, cut into wedges
- 3 tablespoons + 4 tablespoons (separately) Olive oil
- 1 tablespoon ½ teaspoon (separately) Oregano, fresh or dried
- 1 teaspoon + ½ teaspoon (separately) Parsley, dried
- Ground black pepper, paprika, red pepper flakes and sea salt to taste

Instructions:

1. Combine 3 tablespoons of olive oil and cubes of chicken in a large bowl. Stir in 1 teaspoon of salt, 1 teaspoon of parsley, 1 tablespoon of oregano, 7 cloves of crushed garlic, zest and juice of 1 lemon. Add paprika, black pepper, and cherry tomatoes. Stir very thoroughly. Set it aside for a while.

2. In the meanwhile prepare garlic sauce. Combine 2 cloves of crushed garlic, zest, and juice of the second lemon, ½ teaspoon of parsley, ½ teaspoon of oregano, 4 tablespoons of olive oil, salt, black pepper and red pepper flakes. Whisk together to make a smooth sauce.

3. Set the grill to medium-high heat and soak bamboo skewers in the water for 5-10 minutes.

4. Skewer meat and tomatoes onto bamboo skewers and grill them for several minutes both sides. The meat should turn golden-brown and become tender. Check its readiness with a point of a knife. Repeat until you cook all meat skewers.

5. Pour the garlic sauce over the cooked meat and tomatoes. Garnish with lemon wedges. Serve immediately.

GARLIC CAJUN SHRIMP NOODLES

Ingredients:

- 15-18 large and fresh Shrimps, peeled and deveined
- 2 Zucchinis, large and previously spiralized
- 3 tablespoons + 1 tablespoon (separately) Extra Virgin Olive Oil
- 1 Red bell pepper, cut lengthwise
- 1 Onion, sliced
- 3 cloves Garlic, minced or crushed
- 1 teaspoon Garlic powder
- 1 teaspoon Onion powder
- 1 teaspoon Paprika, ground
- ⅛ teaspoon Chile pepper, ground
- ⅛ teaspoon Red pepper flakes
- ½ teaspoon Sea salt

Instructions:

Make Cajun seasoning combining paprika, red pepper flakes, chile pepper, garlic powder, onion powder and sea salt. Mix up with detailed shrimps.

Heat 3 tablespoons of olive oil in the frying pan. Add garlic, red bell pepper and onion. Smoother at medium-low heat for 4 minutes.

Increase heat to medium-high and add Cajun seasoned shrimps. Cook stirring for 4 minutes. Turn off the heat and leave covered.

In the meanwhile take another frying pan, set medium-low heat, and add the remaining 1 tablespoon of olive oil. Add spiralized zucchinis and smoother for 5 minutes.

Transfer zucchini noodles to the serving bowls. Cover them with Cajun seasoned shrimps and veggies. Dinner is ready!

GRILLED PORTOBELLO MUSHROOMS

Ingredients:

- 4 Portobello mushrooms, large-sized
- 6 cloves Garlic, unpeeled
- 1 tablespoon Dijon mustard (alcohol-free)
- ⅓ cup Balsamic vinegar
- 2 tablespoons + ¾ cup + 2 tablespoons (all separately) Olive oil
- Sea salt to taste

Instructions:

1. Preheat the oven to 350 F and preheat the grill at medium-high heat.

2. Toss unpeeled garlic cloves with a pinch of salt and 2 tablespoons Olive oil. Wrap all garlic cloves into tinfoil and place in preheated oven for 25 minutes.

3. In the meanwhile take another ¾ cup olive oil, pour it into a medium bowl and add mustard and balsamic vinegar. Whisk thoroughly. Set this dressing aside.

4. Take another medium bowl and add the last 2 tablespoons olive oil, mushrooms, and salt. Toss the mushrooms and transfer them to

grill. Cook for 4 minutes stem-side up and later 4 minutes stem-side down.

5. Transfer the mushrooms to the oven and cook for 10-15 minutes more, until tender. Check tenderness with the knife tip. Remove the mushrooms and sprinkle each with another pinch of salt.

6. Unwrap garlic from the foil and whisk it to the dressing that you have set aside in step 3. Transfer the mushrooms to the serving plate and pour the dressing all over it. Now serve.

GRILLED ROSEMARY LAMB CHOPS

Ingredients:

- 4 Lamb chops, thickness about ¾-inch
- 1 teaspoon Rosemary
- ½ teaspoon Thyme leaves
- 2 teaspoons Garlic powder
- 2 tablespoons Extra virgin olive oil
- 4 tablespoons fresh Lemon juice
- Chili pepper and sea salt to taste

Instructions:

1. Make the marinade by mixing lemon juice, olive oil, garlic powder, thyme, rosemary, chili pepper, and salt.

2. Lamb chops should be marinated in closed pan or zip lock bag for at least 2 hours and up to 24 hours.

3. 30 minutes prior to grilling take the pan or bag with lamb and marinade off the refrigerator. Let it warm up to the room temperature.

4. Grill for about 4 or 5 minutes each side.

GROUND BEEF AND VEGETABLE SOUP

Ingredients:

- 2 ½ lbs. ground Beef
- 3 cups Beef broth
- 2 Sweet potatoes, chopped roughly
- 3 Tomatoes, large and diced
- 4 Carrots, sliced
- 1 large Onion, minced
- 3 Green bell peppers, deseeded and chopped
- 2 Celery stalks, minced
- 3 tablespoons Tomato paste
- 3 cloves Garlic, crushed
- 1 teaspoon Chili powder
- ½ teaspoon Oregano
- 1 tablespoon Olive oil
- Salt and ground black pepper to taste

Instructions:

1. Stir-fry garlic and onion in a medium-sized oiled skillet over medium-high heat for 2-3 minutes. Add celery, tomato paste and ground beef. Cook stirring occasionally for 5-7 minutes until meat turns brown.

2. Take a large saucepan and combine beef broth, potatoes, tomatoes, carrot, bell pepper, chili powder, and oregano. Pour contents of the skillet and stir. Bring to a boil, reduce heat and let it simmer.

3. Simmer for 15-20 when potatoes get tender. Check their softness with the fork. Taste it hot or warm.

CROCK-POT CHICKEN CACCIATORE

Ingredients:

- 3 lbs. Chicken, boneless and skinless, cut into bite-size pieces
- 6 oz. Button mushrooms, chopped
- 12 oz. Tomato paste
- ½ cup White wine vinegar
- 1 Bell pepper (green is better here), minced
- 1 Yellow onion, minced
- 4 cloves Garlic, crushed
- 1 tablespoon Basil leaves
- 1 tablespoon dried Oregano
- 3 tablespoons Olive oil
- Ground Black pepper, Red pepper flakes, and Sea salt to taste

Instructions:

1. Put minced onion inside the crock-pot first and cover with chicken pieces.

2. In a large bowl combine mushrooms, olive oil, tomato paste, white wine vinegar, bell pepper, crushed garlic. Sprinkle with basil leaves, pepper flakes, salt, black pepper and dried oregano. Stir thoroughly.

3. Pour the mixture from the large bowl over the chicken and onion.

4. Cook on high heat for about 3-3.5 hours. Check the readiness with the point of a knife.

GRILLED BEEF TENDERLOIN STEAK WITH GARLIC DRESSING AND AVOCADO

Ingredients:

- 2 x 5oz. Beef tenderloin steaks
- 1 Avocado, halved lengthwise, seeded and peeled
- 1 tablespoon + 1 tablespoon (separately) Olive oil
- 2 cloves Garlic, not minced, only peeled
- 1 Shallot, minced
- Ground black pepper and sea salt to taste

Instructions:

1. Before you start, steaks should rest at room temperature. So make sure to remove them from the fridge at least half hour in advance.

2. Preheat oven to 375 F and preheat grill to 500 F. Cover the baking dish with tinfoil.

3. Season steaks generously with salt and pepper.

4. In a small bowl mix 1 tablespoon of olive oil, shallot, and peeled garlic cloves. Add salt and pepper and cook it in the oven for 25 minutes. Then transfer the mix to the food processor, add 1 more tablespoon of olive oil and mash it completely. Pour this puree into a small bowl and cover to keep warm.

5. Grill the steaks for 2-3 minutes each side and let them rest for at least 5 minutes.

6. Meanwhile, grill halved avocado, round side up, for 3 minutes.

7. Transfer steaks to the serving plate and sprinkle with warm garlic dressing. Add grilled avocado and serve.

ASIAN TURKEY PATTY LETTUCE WRAPS

Ingredients:

- 1 lb. Turkey, ground
- 12 Lettuce leaves (choose butter lettuce or romaine lettuce if available), washed
- 1 large Cucumber, matchstick-shape cut
- 1 tablespoon Ginger root, freshly grated
- 2 cloves Garlic, crushed
- 1 cup Mint, leaves of
- 3 tablespoons Fish sauce
- 4 tablespoons + 1 tablespoon (separately) Rice vinegar
- 1 teaspoon Coconut aminos
- 1 tablespoon + 1 tablespoon (separately) Sesame oil
- 1 teaspoon + 1 teaspoon (separately) Coconut oil
- ½ teaspoon Red pepper flakes

Instructions:

1. Mix up 4 tablespoons of rice vinegar, 1 tablespoon of sesame oil, fish sauce and pepper flakes. Set aside this Asian sauce.

2. In a large bowl combine ground turkey with crushed garlic and freshly grated ginger. Thoroughly stir in remaining 1 tablespoon of rice vinegar, 1 tablespoon of sesame oil and soy sauce.

3. Add 1 teaspoon of coconut oil to the large skillet and set medium-high heat level.

4. Take a heaped tablespoon of turkey mixture each time to make a small patty, and place it in the skillet. Do not crowd the frying pan. Cook patties in two batches.

5. Lightly brown each side of the patties and turn them to the other side. When both sides are light brown, remove the patties to a large plate.

6. Add another 1 teaspoon of coconut oil and add the second batch of meat.

7. When all patties are ready, transfer 2-3 patties onto each lettuce leaf. Sprinkle meat with the Asian sauce and top with chopped cucumber and the leaves of mint. Ready to eat now!

Conclusion

Eating on a plant-based whole foods have a lot of benefits such as losing weight, avoid food allergens, and feel great about yourself and your body!

I hope, this book recipes helped you with wonderful recipes that are so delightful you won't even understand you're without meat, dairy, from your diet. I hope this whole foods cookbook will become a life changer for you.

Keep your meals exciting by following the recipes and sample meal plan outlined in this book!

CPSIA information can be obtained
at www.ICGtesting.com
Printed in the USA
BVHW041917050819
555124BV00009B/302/P